The Curious Case Of The Shrinking Woman

The simple story of how a normal woman lost some weight and simply made herself feel better.

by Novelist
Kitty O'Day

Copyright @ Kitty O'Day 2013

I struggled with 'baby' weight but eventually found a solution that worked for me.

List Of Contents

Introduction

I am not a scientist or nutritonist, a keep-fit fanatic or a paid celebrity.

I am a Mum of four who has struggled with eating and weight. I have a thyroid condition which made things 'difficult' but then that was sorted and other things happened to make life and food go astray.

When all that was sorted and I felt like me and I was happy. I don't think as a twenty something you fully appreciate your flattish tummy and gravity defying boobs.

Then you have children; and boy does the laws of gravity and elastasine change. What I wouldn't do for an apronectomy now.

So, I am just a normal Mum who wanted to feel like me again. My change was very quick to those watching, once I found the way of eating that suited me I 'melted'. Since this so many people have asked me to write down what I can eat, what I don't and to share my recipes. So here is the stuff I can eat, the food I like to cook and how I have done and are still doing.

I hope what I have discovered can help other people feel just like they want to feel again.

The Background.

Sometimes you just have to be ready to do something life changing. However much you think you want it, or your brain says it is what you have to do. The trick is to be utterly determined; have every cell in your body demanding change. Then you can succeed. But only with the lingering taste of fear reminding you what it is like to do nothing to help yourself.

In a time that I have almost forgotten, I weighed between 8 and a quarter and 8 and a half stone. After years of suffering with an undiagnosed thyroid condition and the weight problems that this brings; everything was under control.

I have been the same weight for a good few years. I am only small 5ft 2 if I really stand straight so I was in 'proportion' with myself, not skinny, not fat- just me.

Then I had my first child, which was a surprise even 10 years later that I am still getting over, but that, as they say is another story. I put on nearly 3 stone. Argh!

But, as you supposed, I started a GI diet which was great. This and doing up the house we had bought, gave me plenty of opportunity for exercise. Scrapping the wallpaper from walls is hard work- it gives you muscles and gets rid of bingo wings.

I lost just over a stone; brilliant!

Then I discovered I was pregnant again! Another shock....both children 'happened' while I was on the pill, so you can understand I feel overwhelmed by motherhood even now.

So well, Ok, I thought. It will be fine after this one has popped out; still loads to do on the house and the GI diet we were still trying to stick to, was still good.

Then work, and running about in general kept things on an even keel- but I was still overweight.

Two more children later, and I was edging nearer 5 stone heavier than I should have been. I refused to buy any clothes that were more than a dress size 18/20 out of sheer embarrassment. I would just plonk a huge XXL jumper of my husband's on. He was getting bigger too.

When I realised that I didn't want any more children; two emergency c-sections, fitting in IT and a baby in NICU for a bit sort of puts you off, I decided I had to lose the weight.

I started a new job, which meant I ran around a kitchen for four hours every day, so that gave my body a new shape, but not really losing much of the extra. I was back in a size 18, but still way over 12 probably nearer, if I admit it- 13 stone.

When I was at the doctor's he stopped me taking the pill because he said I was 'too fat.' He is very blunt; but I'm Northern, so quite used to it.

'Oh bugger,' says I, 'I have been trying to lose weight but it is proving hard, can you suggest anything?'

'Stop eating too much.'

'Eh, be-buggery doctor, I'd a never thought a-that.'

I went away. A little pissed off.

So I decide to do the most sensible thing and started to reduce calories. I am a cook and a bit of a foodie, I enjoy a balance to my diet. I love vegetables and fruit. I am a bit of a pudding-face, but I can be very restrained when I need to be. Too much always spoils the enjoyment for me; I much prefer a little bit of something naughty.

So I kept a food diary.

I went from 1800 calories, which I thought was what a woman needed, down to 1600. I did this for a month or so, then reduced again as nothing was happening.

Now before you start, I wasn't just eating 1600 calories of chocolate and crisps and other rubbish. My husband cooks from scratch, wonderful Guyana curries (no cream in these of course) lots of veggies and couscous and whole grains. I devised some really delicious recipes with sweet chilli, beans pulses and roasted vegetables. All the things that are advertised as good for your system. Plenty of fibre from all sources, some protein, a little carbohydrate, some dairy, vitamins and minerals.

But I just did not seem to lose any weight this time.

It was July and I was, quite frankly getting a little depressed. I was down to eating between 500-600 calories a day and I weighed myself everyday for three weeks and not an ounce had disappeared.

I was size 18 and at that point 12st, 8 lbs in the nip.

I looked on the NHS website, which, if you put in your weight and size it will tell you where you are on the 'underweight', 'ok', 'over-weight,' 'obese', or 'morbidly obese' scale.

For my height, I should be between 8 and a half, and 9 and a half stone-ish, according to the chart.

But at 12 and a half, I was well into the 'obese' section. My body-fat ratio was huge. In short I was a weight-related disaster waiting to happen; with my paternal family all dying at 65 due to heart conditions and some having diabetes, I needed to do something.

So I plucked up the courage and swallowed the bitter taste of embarrassment, and booked an appointment with my doctor's surgery. I saw a locum....

I calmly told her that I had been restricting calories, I even took my food diary in with me. I asked if there was something else that I could be doing because I clearly was doing something wrong.

She snapped back at me, 'I'm not going to give you any drugs you know!'

'But I don't want any drugs.'

'They don't work. At my last surgery we did a survey and found they don't work at all. I'm not going to give you any.'

'Well that's grand. I didn't ask for any and don't want to take any drugs. I need help and advice... By your own NHS website I am obese. I need practical help, not drugs.'

'Have you tried exercise, it is the only thing that works?'

'I have a family, and I work in a job that does not allow me to sit down. I run around for 4 hours every day. My husband leaves the house at 7.20 and doesn't get home till just before 7pm; where exactly could I fit in a gym visit?'

'That is the only thing; join a gym.'

'I'm a bankrupt. I haven't got enough money to eat and heat the house at the same time, I cannot justify joining a gym!'

The consultation came to a close.

Depression was hitting; sort of understandable.

I pulled myself together and a few weeks later I booked another appointment with my own doctor, or at the very least not the locum.

I saw the other resident doctor, one who is not known for his bedside manor either; I put on my best 'don't give me any shit,' face and went in to see him.

I explained that I was told to join a gym and I don't and never have wanted to take drugs. I showed him my food diary.

'Look watch the carbs, not the calories and you'll see results. Some people just don't respond to calorie diets, you're just one of those. I have been on a low carb diet because eating less calories was not working and I have lost 5 stone. The moment I ignored the carbohydrates I put half a stone back on. Try it.'

Halleluyah! A sensible answer.

'Is there a plan?' I asked in all innocence.

'I'm not going to give you a plan because you won't stick to it, you're a cook you'll just do your own thing anyway, so don't eat anymore than 20 grams of carbs a day and see how you get on. Now go.'

So I went away, and looked at all the things I had been eating.

Lots of healthy things, but a quite high in carbohydrates. Beans and pulses-carb city.

Anything with flour in- off the scale. Rice and potatoes- ha!

So I had a re-think.

The next day was tuff. I cannot have a bowl of cereal (most with milk are about 30 carbs) no toast (one slice approx 20 carbs) and fruit yoghurt about 20 carbs per small pot.

Mmmm.

Day One, Week One.

Breakfast? What the hell do I eat?

Then it came to me, we have chickens; they lay eggs- egg salad.

Two boiled eggs, a big handful of salad leaves and a blob of Mayo (personal taste), approx 174 calories for the eggs, 20 for the salad and 20 for the mayo.

Carbohydrates; nil, .25, and .25

Job done.

I have recently read that eating eggs in a morning is good for you. Something to do with the combination of fats and protein in the eggs keep you feeling fuller for longer. Well all I can say is that it works for me.

I felt good- although it would take me months to get my head around eating a salad for breakfast every morning. It just seems so un-natural.

A good lunch for the first day;

Chicken and bacon lasagna

	Calories	Carbohydrates
2oz strong cheese	200	trace
Chicken Breast x2	400	trace
Bacon x2	100	trace
Condensed soup for sauce	120	22.6
Mushrooms	20	trace
Spinach	20	0.5
1 Leek	38	9.0
	898	31.1

This makes about three portions that my husband and I could eat, then the spare portion would be for my dinner the next day. Having something ready prepared at dinner time makes dieting so much easier.

299cal, 10.3 carbs per portion- ish.

Trim any fat from the chicken and bacon, then fry off the diced chicken breasts and bacon. Throw in the mushrooms and spinach (I often use frozen for convenience).

Mix in the condensed soup for the sauce.

Use the leek as a pasta substitute. With thanks to 'The Hairy Biker's' for this brilliant tip, (and for helping my husband lose 4 stone with their brilliant book).

Trim the top and bottom and slice down the leek on one side. Un-roll the layers and separate them out. In another pan, boil some water. Plunge the layers into the water to blanch and 'flatten' the leeks.

Put the mixture in an oven proof dish, layering it up using the leek just as you would if using pasta.

I like to sprinkle cheese on the top.

Bake in oven until the cheese has melted and is bubbly and browning around the edges.

Then a quick dinner.

Sliced an aubergine in half. Scooped out a 'channel' Then filled it with mushrooms, courgette cubes and the scooped out bit cut into cubes. Then a table spoon of sweet chilli sauce.

Roasted in oven till done.

 Approx 5 Carbs

I cannot give up drinking tea and I need a little milk with it so I have to allow about 5 carbs per day for 100ml of 1% fat milk (Semi).

That usually makes me about four cups.

So Day One;

	Carbs
Breakfast	.5
Lunch	10.3
Dinner	5.0
Milk in Tea	5.0
Total	**20.5 approx.**

Day Two.

Breakfast

	Carbs
Egg x 2	0.0
Salad & Mayo	0.5

Lunch

Yesterday's Chicken & Bacon Lasagna	10.3

Dinner

Prawns, Garlic & Spinach	0.5

Drinks

Milk for Tea	5.0
Total	**16.0**

Day Three
Breakfast

	Carbs
Egg x 2	00.0
Salad & Mayo	0.5

Lunch

Minced Beef	5.6

Dinner

Soup	0.8
Salad	0.5

Drinks

Milk for Tea	5.0
Total	**10.4**

Day Four
Breakfast

	Carbs
Eggs x 2	00.0
Salad & Mayo	0.5

Lunch

Cheese & Ham Salad	1.5
Half oz Pecan nuts	0.75

Dinner

Cassaulet	13.6

Drinks

	5.0
Total	**21.4**

Day Five

Breakfast

Eggs x 2	00.0
Salad & Mayo	0.5

Lunch

Roasted Squash, Olive   3.0

oil & pine nut salad

(A friend made this; roasted squash and pine nuts, when cold tossed in some salad leaves and drizzled with oil, s& p to taste.)

Dinner

Fish Pie   4.5

Drinks

Milk for Tea   5.0

Total   **13.0**

Day Six Saturday

Breakfast	Carbs	
Bacon x 2		00.0
Salad & Mayo	0.5	

Lunch

	Carbs
Butchers Beef Burger	2.0
Roasted Cougette, aubergine	1.5
Salad	0.5

Dinner

	Carbs
Chicken wrapped in Bacon	0.5
Roasted Vegetables	4.5
Half oz Pecan Nuts	0.75

Drinks

	Carbs
Milk for Tea	5.0
Sparkling Water	1.2

Total	**15.95**

Day Seven Sunday- Naughty Day!

Breakfast	Carbs
Egg x 2	00.0
Salad	00.5
Dressing, a drizzle	00.5

(Wholegrain Mustard, Olive Oil, White wine vinegar, S&P to taste)

Lunch

Roast Beef	00.5
Roasted courgette, aubergine, a few carrot sticks,	2.0
Gravy	1.0
Peas	1.0
Broccoli	2.0
Slither of Pudding with cream,	10.0

Dinner

50g/2oz cheese	00.0
Slice of ham	00.2
Pickle, small blob	2.0

Drinks

Milk for tea	5.0
Sparkling flavoured water	1.2

Total Carbs for the day,	**25.9 ish.**

Not terribly exciting, but practical and tasty, and yes I lost 7lbs in the first week!

All 'wind an' w'ater' as my granny would say, but I felt less bloated and very positive.

I went to a family wedding, still a size 18, but my clothes were not tight and I felt fantastic; at last, something that worked for me and worked around my lifestyle.

I don't know for sure how this all works. The doctor said something about carbohydrates acting as 'glue' to help the calories stick. Lowering carbs, means there is less for the fat to stick too.

He also said the recommended 2000 calories a day for me, been small would be way too much. A more sensible 12-1500 would be more appropriate to maintain weight.

I have since found from reading on the sides of packets (you do have to do this a lot) that the recommended is 230 carbohydrates per day.

I think I would be the size of a house if I ate that many... I don't think I have ever eaten that much. But there are 'good' carbs and 'bad' carbs. I think we can all guess that anything processed, chocolate and flour included are probably not the best things to eat too much of on a regular basis.

We are all well aware that vegetables are good, even the ones high in carbohydrates. At first you have to watch out for carrots, sweetcorn anything grown under the ground. They are ok to reintroduce when you want your weight to level off.

Leave off the fruit and fruit juices for a bit, then re-introduce when needed; but you will be surprised that some veg, like Broccoli can have the same vits and mins as a piece of fruit. So if you do your research on-line you can pick and choose the best thing for you.

It is all about balance- as we all know- I'm not going to patronise anyone, just tell you what I am doing to lose this baby weight of mine.

For a diet to work for me I need to be organised, because I am a bit of a disorganised, busy person in general. So things have to be easy.

I cook the main meal with portions to spare, so I have something for the next day's lunch. I can freeze extra portions because we all get busy and a bit lazy some days.

If I am not organised for whatever reason I just end up grabbing something quick which inevitably means 'full of carbohydrates'. Then the diet goes bump.

So my advice whatever diet you want to follow is; be organised and plan ahead- then it will work.

Next are some of my recipes for you to mix and match, all guides are approximate and will vary upon brands and size of food, but as a guide please....

ENJOY!

Recepies

Cassaulet

	Carbohydrates	Calories
Good Quality Sausages x 6	6.0	900
Chicken Breasts, trimmed x 4	00.0	800
Gammon, trimmed One	00.0	400
Celery a stick	00.0	10
Onion	9.0	50
Tomatos (tin)	18.0	104
Red wine, 125ml	10.0	130
Stock	1.0	20
Carrots x 2	2.0	50
Mixed Beans- one tin	36.0	226
Garlic, Chilli flakes, Bay, Thyme, S&P		
Total	82.0	2690

Divide into 6 portions   448 Cals

13.6 Carbs

Use an oven proof/hob proof pan. I have a cast iron big thing that does the job brilliantly.

Quickly fry off the sausages, remove and fry off chicken and gammon. Remove. Then fry onion and celery with the garlic. When brown, return meat to dish.

Add the wine and the stock (made from cubes) add the chilli flakes, bay leaf, some thyme, salt and pepper to taste.

Add carrots, chopped small into batons and the rinsed tin of mixed beans.

Give it a good stir and when it is bubbling put in the oven on medium for at least an hour, but for the best results leave on low for a few hours.

This dish tastes even better warmed up for lunch the next day. It freezes well for when you don't have the time or inclination to cook, but still want a nice meal.

Beef Bourginion

	Carbohydrates	Calories
Beef lean, about 1kg	00.0	1200
A desert spoon of flour	11.4	15
Oil	00.0	100
Small onions/ or chop into Quarters- 4oz ish	12.0	50
Button Mushrooms/or chop Into quarters 2oz ish	0.5	20
Bacon rashers x 4 trimmed and chopped	00.0	200
125ml of Burgundy Wine	10.0	130
200ml ish of stock	1.0	20
Garlic, x 2 Bay, Thyme, S&P Garlic pepper.		
Total	34.9	1735
Divide into six portions	**5.8 Carbs**	**289 Cals**

Put the flour onto a plate, then add the salt and pepper (I like freshly ground sea salt and black pepper).

Roll the beef into the flour while you heat the oil and garlic pepper in a cast iron pan than can be used on the top and in the oven. Fry off the beef. Remove then fry off the garlic, onions and bacon.

Return the beef. Put in the wine and stock (I use a cube but always add a teaspoon of bovril for taste). Add the mushrooms, bay and thyme. Keep stirring to prevent it sticking.

Stir in the rest of the flour, this can sometimes form 'blobs', try to stir in well, but it is not the end of the world.

Put in the oven for at least an hour and half, but again the lower and longer the better. This tastes even better the next day and is again, great to freeze.

Basic Minced Beef

	Carbohydrates	Calories
Minced beef 500g	00.0	600
Onions 4oz	12.0	50
Tomatoes- half a tin	9.0	52
Stock, plus Bovril 1 teaspoon	0.5	20
Frozen spinach cube	0.5	10
Mushrooms 2oz	0.5	20
Herbs to taste, Garlic Pepper		
Total	22.5	752
Divide into Four portions	**5.6 Carbs**	**188 Cals**

This makes a great bowl for lunch.

Fry off the mince and onions in a little oil and garlic pepper. Add the tomatoes, spinach and mushrooms, then stir in the stock and the bovril. Add herbs to taste, a bay leaf for depth, a little basil perhaps? Whatever you like. Cook on low, or in the oven for about 30-40 mins.

Then come tomorrow use the left- overs, here are a few ideas.

Scoop out a marrow (4oz of marrow equals 2 carbs) roast it a little then fill with a portion of the mince and return to the oven. Very, very, filling and delicious.

Or add a few kidney beans (a dessert spoon would be about 3-4 carbs) some chilli flakes and mixed spice.

Garlic Prawns and Spinach

	Carbohydrates	Calories
Oil, olive is best	00.0	200
Prawns	00.0	200
Fresh Spinach	1.0	30
Garlic, Garlic Pepper		
Total	1.0	430

Divide into two   **215 Cals**
         0.5 Carbs

Really simple supper. Heat the oil, throw in the garlic and garlic pepper. Next the prawns. Cook these until they have curled and turned grey. Just before the prawns are ready throw in the spinach leaves.

I like this either in a roasted red pepper (5 carbohydrates), or add some salami or chorizo. (fry this a little in the oil first, then position on a plate. Tip over the garlic prawns when they are done).

Fish pie.

	Carbohydrates	Calories
White fish	00.0	200
Prawns	00.0	160
Boiled Egg x 1	00.0	77
Knob of Butter	00.0	50
Mushrooms, 200g	1.5	100
Veg stock	0.5	20
Garlic Pepper, Salt,		
Teaspoon whole grain mustard	0.5	20
Peas 2oz	5.0	50
Spinach	0.5	20
Cheese, 2oz	00.0	200
Total	9.0	1017

Divide into two portions **505.5 Cals**
4.5 Carbs

First make the sauce. Fry the garlic pepper, wholegrain mustard and S&P, with the mushrooms. Blitz with a blender. Add the stock, till you have a thick sauce.

Boil the egg, cool and shell.

Find a oven-proof dish, fill with the fish (chop) and the prawns, spinach, chopped up egg, peas and any herbs you fancy (I like a little Sage, or sometimes Basil). Pour over the sauce. Sprinkle with cheese and put in the oven for about an hour on medium, or until the cheese is darkened and bubbling.

This makes huge portions, you may want to divide into three; Yum.

Garlic mushroom soup.

	Carbohydrates	Calories
Mushrooms 500g	2.5	250
Garlic	00.0	20
1 teaspoon wholegrain mustard	0.5	50
Garlic pepper		
Veg stock	0.5	20
Worcester sauce, splash		
Basil, oregano		
Total	3.5	340

Divide into four Portions   **85 Cals**
0.8 Carbs

Fry the garlic pepper, garlic, wholegrain mustard and the chopped up mushrooms in a pan. Add a splash of Worcester sauce and herbs. Add the stock.

Blend everything together, add more water if needed, or a little drizzle of cream.

Beef In Gravy

	Carbohydrates	Calories
Beef 500g	00.0	600
Onion 2oz	6.0	25
Garlic Pepper, Basil, Chilli powder half a teaspoon		
Stock x 2 cubes	0.5	20
1 teaspoon Bovril	0.5	20
Mushrooms, 2oz	0.5	20
Spinach	0.5	20
Peas 2oz	5.0	50
Total	13.0	755

Divide into three large portions!

251.7 Cals

4.4 Carbs

Use a cast iron pan that can go in the oven.

Brown the onion in a little butter till soft, add the beef and garlic pepper (you may need a little extra oil). Rip the mushrooms, throw in the peas. Add the stock, bovril and basil.

Put in the oven on low for two hours.

Wonderful as a 'soup-type' meal the next day.

Chicken & Bacon

This is my version of a kiev.

	Carbohydrates	Calories
Chicken breast	00.0	200
Bacon x2 trimmed	00.0	100
Knob of butter	00.0	20
Garlic paste and mixed herbs		
Total	00.0 Carbs	320 Cals

Mix the softened butter with the garlic paste and herbs. Slice the chicken breast down the side and fill with the butter. Wrap the bacon around the chicken. Wrap the whole thing (or as many as you are making) in tin foil and place on a deep oven tray.

Pop in oven on medium for about 30- 40 mins.

Serve with salad or roasted vegetables, for example; cubes of aubergine and courgette, squash (not too much) and a few carrot sticks.

Be Prepared- The Story So Far.

If I am re-heating something, I add more herbs or spices to change the flavour a little. It usually starts off mild and then gets spicier.

I don't waste anything- left-overs are great. If you are left with a tasty stock when all the meat and vegetables are eaten, put it in the fridge. It will keep for three or four days in total. Or freeze. Just remember the golden rule; always re-heat thoroughly. It must be piping hot. That is the only piece of professional advice I can give you.

Most of my winter meals are one pot wonders. Meat and veg, spices and herbs, the essential garlic pepper and stock. Then throw in the bottom of a low oven and ignore for a few hours. Minimal washing up (who needs more work?). Simple to prepare, even when children are about firing five hundred questions at you, and the long cooking melts even the cheapest cuts of meat.

I do love my veg, beans and pulses. But at first this diet did not allow that many carbs, just a spoon of beans in things, rather than using the whole tin for the meal.

But.

...a month later I weighed 11 stone 6.5 lbs.

So after the first initial madness of losing 7lbs, the loss slowed to a sensible few pounds a week.

After the second month I was 10 stone 10 lbs.

I learnt to write everything down, then you can see what you are eating and it puts you off eating too much as it is there in black and white; your sins staring at you!

Month three- 10 stone 3lbs and I discovered I have a cracking pair of legs! I have always hated my legs, always worn skirts to the floor. But maybe it was just I have always had forty year old legs, and I'm just growing into them. Give me another year or two and they'll be grand.

End of month four, 9 stone 8 lbs Yeah! Within range but I wanted to be slap bang in the middle of the recommended for me, so 9 stone was my goal.

Then Christmas happened....

Oh come on what is a girl to do when there are chocolate brasils in the shops? Leave them there to go off? Of course not!

So from the middle of December till the end of February I had a bit of a diet rest. I needed a break for counting and looking at packets.

I got back into it though, as I was not going to let all that hard work go to waste. At a size 12 I needed to buy new clothes, that shock horror I actually looked good in and that I wanted to wear. Not just big tents that covered everything or my husband's fleeces.

However the down side? Well my husband thought I was having an affair which is typical dick head man logic. I couldn't possibly be losing weight for myself...or shock horror for him! To look like me again, be confident and positive. But that is men for you. A bit dim.

I kept trying, but someone bought 'Curiously Cinnamon' cereal squares which are so tempting to eat out of the box. They are the perfect combination of sugar and cinnamon. And there is one thing I love just as much as chocolate nuts it is cinnamon.

I know restraint should be applied in this circumstance- but hell? Come on? Did the devil himself sneak into the pantry with that temptation? Bugger!

So some weeks I put on a few pounds, then I was good and lost a few.

I have stayed about 9.6 - 9.8 since then.

Now March has started and I need to attack this with gusto again. I am too small to be a size 12 but just too big to be a 10. I need to either put a little on (my jeans fall down as I walk) or lose that extra (buy more clothes. I might even start wearing dresses again, ooer missus).

I think I am going to lose.

However I mourn the disappearance of my boobs. I woke one morning and they had gone- it was quite a shock. I found what was left quivering under my arm pits, seems the boob goblin got'em in the night. Damn.

I have always worn a low cleavage to distract from every other physical inadequacy, what the hell am gonna do now I don't know? Answers on a postcard please.

Snacking is hard to avoid for me. When I'm being good I am really good, but when I'm not I am naughty.

It is habit sometimes, comfort eating; craving carbohydrates to ease the mind, or boredom.

And quite frankly every woman needs chocolate about 12 times a year and it is

only a fool or a madman who would stand between the two.

This is hard work. Being good, when you don't feel like it- but I have to. I have to be me again. It is all well and good being a mum, wouldn't change it for the world, but I have to be reminded that I am a separate person too.

It is the end of March and I am still trying to lose this half stone. I have started to comfort eat, which is a disaster. It is that 4 o'clock low that starts the main binge off. I have never binged on food like this, especially not sweets and choc, but that is depression for you.

I haven't put any weight on, but I really need to start losing again, just to put me in my weight zone rather than hovering around the edge. All too easy to fall off.

April has started and I have put on 2lbs- 9.9.

I have started back at normal work. I am a school cook, where although I am surrounded by food I am not allowed to eat, wonderful puddings and custard; this is not the problem. I can resist.

It is after when I come home and I start to think.

Thinking should be banned.

Thinking of all the things that are going wobbly, that I just don't know what, or how, to make it alright again.

And I am trying to go back to university- to retrain- hit the re-start button. And that is so bloody infuriating. I have been fighting with the collage since July about coming back. Until last month, they still would not acknowledge that I existed.

Bloody admin!

So I rang up the main campus and spoke to a wonderfully helpful man called Daniel, who found me within a five minute conversation.

So I passed this on.

Nearly the end of April and I still cannot get through to uni. Bloody art departments.

May the first! (Oh that sounds a bit 'Star wars'; May 1st?)

I am 9.6, and hanging on in. The weather is better and I have decided to have more salads. A salad for breakfast and dinner, then a main meal.

I find cooking low carb very easy now so the meals are not the problem, it is comfort eating that is doing for me.

Or being so busy, then not eating anything for dinner. I get the munchies and of course like everyone else, just reach for something convenient and easy. Killer.

So after a week of salads and trying hard, but falling of the diet-wagon occasionally, I am this week 9.6, on average. I say 'average' because what you wear affects your weight. You do not realise how heavy a cardigan is, or a pair of jeans are.

May 4th. 9.6. All good so far, but a couple of chocolate Hobnobs pulled me off the wagon this time. Aaghh, bloody tasty confectionary.

May 5th. 9.5 in jeans- OK, roast dinner with Spotty Dotty ice cream and a slither of choc. Healthy tea-time. Let see if this makes a difference for tomorrow's weigh-in.

May 6th. Forgot to weight in, I was tucking into a bacon and black pudding salad for breakfast that distracted me. (about 0.25 carbs for the black pudding, so healthy too.)

I know, most of you are now curling your face at the thought of black pudding, but it was a treat when I was young- stealing a bit of Dad's black pudding.

Aye daint know, you can teck the girl owt-a Yorksha, but yeh caint teck the Yorksha owt-t girl.

May 7th. Bloody 9.8. What the hell happened? The fat fairy sticks it back on in the night when I'm not looking, that's what!

May 8th. 9.7. Bloody bungy this is.

May 9th. 9.9. :-(

Got depressed and had a hobnob and some crisps. I do feel very low.

Random Tips

Gin has virtually no carbs. Yeah!

Tonic has too many- oh well straight gin it is then.

Or to be more sensible and socially acceptable, water it down with flavoured sparkling water. Tastes nice and refreshing and is very low. (approx 0.6 for 250ml)

Try to avoid wine and beer.

Nuts are a great snack, but look on the packet as some are higher in carbs than others. I like Pecans to snack on- but I must admit, I love roasted, and salted peanuts- which are not that low.

Cream is good and low in carbohydrates. Custard sadly isn't.

Avoid sitting down with a cup of tea and a biscuit- one always leads to five.

I get a real sugar low about 4pm, so I need a snack. Usually it is nuts, sometimes cheese or a slice of ham. My doctor said I could have a few squares of really high percentage chocolate (90%) but it is too bitter for me.

Cut up cucumber, celery stick or maybe a little carrot, or any other healthy, nibbly thing and keep them in the fridge for emergency snacking.

Terry's chocolate orange, as far as sticking to a diet is concerned is the work of the devil. Dieting over Christmas is hopeless; just aim not to put any on over the given period.

I am hopelessly addicted to nuts. I could not live with anyone who was allergic; and if I did they would have to work long weekends away every now and then so I could secretly indulge. If they came home early, they would probably find me catatonic in a bath of chocolate nuts.

I need help.

Lists Of Some Of The Things That Are Good To Eat.

Lean meat, trace-0.4 per good slice.

Most meat, minced or diced is either trace or very small carb value. So meat is good! But don't over-dose on protein it can do funny things to you- apparently.

Egg-	**trace!**	
1 pepper		**4.8g**
½ tin of chopped tomatoes		**0.6g**
Marrow		**2.0g**
Mushrooms, 100g,		**0.4g**
Small apple		**11.2g**
Aubergine		**2.8g**
Sweetcorn, 100g		**17.9g**
Spinach, 100g		**0.5g**
Broccoli, 100g		**1.1g**
Collie, 100g		**2.1g**
Peas, 100g		**0.7g**
Onion, 100g 8.4g = 25g		**2.1g**
White fish, 80g portion	**trace!**	
Prawns,	**trace!**	

Baked beans, ½ tin,	**29.6g**
Adzuki beans, ½ tin,	**24.6g**
Red kidney beans, ½ tin,	**16.2g**
Mixed beans, ½ tin,	**18.3g**

Condensed soup (mushroom) ½ tin,	**9.0g**

Pecan nuts, 14g (½ oz)	**0.75g**
Mixed nuts, 14g(1/2 oz)	**1.61g**
Raisins, 25g	**17.0g**
Chicken in white sauce, ½ tin	**2.2g**

Things You Add To Make It All Taste Nice..

English mustard, 1 tspn		**1.2g**
Wholegrain mustard, 1 tspn	**trace**	(100g =9g, 25g =2.25g)
Soy, per 1g splash		**0.25g**
Sweet chilli dipping sauce 30ml,		**19.3g**
Horseradish sauce,	**trace!**	(25g =2.5g)
Gravy, 70ml		**0.2g**
Oxo stock, 100ml		**0.9g**
Bovril, a good tspn		**0.8g**

Herbs, garlic pepper and such seems to be such a small amount used that I didn't even worry about the carb content! Life is too short for some things.

List of Things To Avoid.

Of course this list contains the things that we all love.

Rice, 100g	**30.6g**
Pasta, (dry weight) 90g	**65.8g**
Egg noodles, per nest	**48.1g**
Couscous, ½ packet	**29.5g**
Plain flour, 100g	**77.7g**
1 tortilla,	**31.8g**
1 slice of bread,	**17.1g**
Sugar, 100g	**100.0g**

So, I'm sorry to say that even if you make a cake then the sugar is pure carb and the flour is about 75% carbohydrate. Drat!

Cream cakes, 100g	**30.0g**
Yoghurts, sm pot	**15.0g**
Cereal, average with semi-skimmed milk,	**28.9g**
Weetabix, 2 with semi milk	**33.2g**

Parsnips, potatoes, oranges and crisps are all really high. Just avoid anything with flour and sugars-even natural sugars for a while. Remember fruit juices are also high in carbohydrates.

My Conclusion.

Go and see your doctor if you want to lose weight. If they suggest low carbohydrate, then I hope these recipes are helpful.

Re-introduce the natural and 'good' carbs when necessary.

Always check the packet, as different brands have different carbohydrate values. I have found that 'low fat' options often have more carbs than the full fat version.

There are many different websites that can give you the carbohydrate values of fruit and vegetables; find the one that you can get on with and 'bookmark' it.

Carbohydrates are vital for a healthy body and system. We do all need them, but there are good carbs and not so good carbs. Research on line, ask your doctor if you can see the nutritionist if your surgery has one; find out what is good for **you** and when to eat them. All meals need to be balanced for **your** needs. That is the hardest part of any diet; keeping the balance right to maintain the size and life you want.

I don't think this is a long term diet, but it changes your eating habits for what I would consider the better. I cannot even face a cereal breakfast anymore- it is salad all the way for me now.

I don't miss rice or pasta with my curries and sauces. I even prefer it. I get to have more of the lovely curry!

I don't eat so many potatoes anymore, I might pinch the odd roasted parsnip- but they all seem so heavy now. I never enjoy it as I did before. So maybe a little less of the heavy carbs could be good for me.

As the old saying goes; 'a little of what you fancy...' not stuff your face with it.

I have reintroduced fruit now, more of the best veg for me, and I know my limits, what I can eat to keep healthy.

Happy dieting! I hope you get to where you need to be, to be happy. I do hope this gives your system a kick start and if your doctor just tells you 'to get on with it', I hope this little book helps.

Will I ever get to 9 stone?

Well, I am trying.

Keep up with progress via my facebook page kitty O'Day and website kittyodayauthor.co.uk

Let me know how you get on with your diet plans so we can all support each other; let's banish this baby weight for good.

www.ingramcontent.com/pod-product-compliance
Lightning Source LLC
Chambersburg PA
CBHW071301280526
45788CB00004B/1797